Hormone Harmony

A Revolutionary Diet Plan for Igniting Fat Loss and Alleviating Hormonal Disturbances

WILLIAMS .C. HARDWICK

TABLE OF CONTENT

7. Green Goddess Detox Soup:

8. Berry Blast Chia Pudding:

9. Grilled Zucchini and Eggplant Roll-Ups:

10. Greek Yogurt and Berry Parfait:

11. Sesame Ginger Tofu Stir-Fry:

12. Cucumber and Mint Infused Water:

13. Sweet Potato and Kale Hash:

14. Almond Butter and Banana Overnight Oats:

15. Garlic and Rosemary Roasted Sweet Potatoes:

16. Spinach and Feta Stuffed Chicken Breast:

17. Berry Spinach Salad with Balsamic Vinaigrette

18. Cabbage and Carrot Slaw with Avocado Dressing:

19. Pesto Zoodles with Cherry Tomatoes:

20. Blueberry Almond Protein Smoothie:

Incorporating Exercise for Maximum Results

The Role of Exercise in Hormonal Balance

High-Intensity Interval Training (HIIT) for Effective Fat Loss

Strength Training for Hormonal Optimization

Guidelines for Effective Strength Training:

INTRODUCTION

In the bustling city of Harmonyville, where the pace of life matched the beat of a thousand footsteps, there existed an enigmatic haven known as "Hormone Harmony." Nestled amidst the verdant hills on the outskirts of town, this revolutionary wellness center was the brainchild of Dr. Amelia Roberts, a visionary endocrinologist with a passion for transforming lives.The air in Hormone Harmony carried whispers of change, and it wasn't just the gentle rustling of leaves or the melodious chirping of birds that created this ethereal symphony. Dr. Roberts had unlocked the secrets of Hormone Harmony, a breakthrough diet plan designed not only to ignite fat loss but also to bring equilibrium to the intricate dance of hormones within the body.As the sun dipped below the horizon, casting a warm glow upon the tranquil haven, eager participants gathered for the unveiling of a program that promised more than just physical transformation. The Hormone Harmony diet plan was a revelation, challenging conventional notions of weight loss by addressing the often-overlooked role of hormones in the process.

Dr. Roberts, a charismatic woman with a twinkle in her eye, stepped onto the stage, exuding an aura of confidence that immediately captivated her audience. She spokc passionately about the interconnected web of hormones governing metabolism, mood, and overall well-being. The crowd listened intently as she unveiled the intricacies of her revolutionary approach, combining scientific precision with a holistic understanding of the body's needs.

Hormone Harmony wasn't just about shedding pounds; it was a journey toward reclaiming vitality and achieving a harmonious balance between body and mind. The program integrated tailored nutrition plans, strategic exercise routines, and mindfulness practices, all meticulously crafted to address individual hormonal imbalances.

As word of Hormone Harmony spread like wildfire, the wellness haven became a beacon of hope for those weary of fad diets and quick fixes. In the heart of Harmonyville, a transformational movement was underway—one that promised not just a slimmer waistline but a reinvigorated life fueled by the power of hormonal harmony. The sun had set, but in the world of Hormone Harmony, a new dawn was on the horizon.

Understanding the Body's Hormonal Landscape

Hormones and Their Impact on Weight

Hormones play a crucial role in regulating various physiological functions within the body, including metabolism and weight management. Understanding how hormones impact weight can provide valuable insights into designing an effective approach to weight loss and overall health. Here's a brief overview of key hormones and their influence on weight:

1. **Insulin:**

   - *Role:* Regulates blood sugar levels by facilitating the absorption of glucose into cells.

   - *Impact on Weight:* High insulin levels, often associated with refined carbohydrate consumption, can lead to increased fat storage. Balancing insulin is essential for effective weight management.

2. **Leptin:**

   - *Role:* Produced by fat cells, leptin signals to the brain when the body has had enough to eat, promoting feelings of fullness.

   - *Impact on Weight:* Leptin resistance can occur, where the brain doesn't respond adequately to leptin signals, leading to overeating and weight gain.

3. **Ghrelin:**

   - *Role:* Known as the "hunger hormone," ghrelin stimulates appetite and promotes the intake of food.

   - *Impact on Weight:* Imbalances in ghrelin levels can result in increased hunger, making it challenging to maintain a healthy weight.

4. **Cortisol:**

   - *Role:* Released in response to stress, cortisol helps the body cope with challenges.

   - *Impact on Weight:* Chronic stress and elevated cortisol levels can lead to increased abdominal fat storage and cravings for unhealthy foods.

5. **Thyroid Hormones (T3 and T4):**

   - *Role:* Regulate metabolism by influencing the rate at which the body burns calories.

   - *Impact on Weight:* Imbalances in thyroid hormones can lead to weight fluctuations, fatigue, and changes in energy levels.

6. **Estrogen and Testosterone:**

   - *Role:* Besides their reproductive functions, these hormones influence body composition and fat distribution.

   - *Impact on Weight:* Hormonal imbalances, such as low estrogen in women or low testosterone in men, can contribute to weight gain and difficulties in losing weight.

7. **Adiponectin:**

   - *Role:* Released by fat cells, adiponectin helps regulate glucose levels and fatty acid breakdown.

   - *Impact on Weight:* Higher levels of adiponectin are associated with better insulin sensitivity and a lower risk of obesity-related diseases.

The Role of Insulin, Cortisol, and Thyroid Hormones in Weight Regulation

1. **Insulin:**

   - *Function:* Insulin is a hormone produced by the pancreas that plays a pivotal role in regulating blood sugar levels. It facilitates the uptake of glucose by cells for energy or storage.

   - *Weight Regulation:* High insulin levels, often triggered by the consumption of refined carbohydrates and sugary foods, promote fat storage. Controlling insulin spikes through a balanced diet can contribute to weight management.

2. **Cortisol:**

   - *Function:* Cortisol, often referred to as the stress hormone, is produced by the adrenal glands in response to stress. It helps the body cope with challenges by mobilizing energy reserves.

- *Weight Regulation:* Chronic stress and consistently elevated cortisol levels can lead to increased abdominal fat storage. Managing stress through relaxation techniques and adequate sleep is crucial for maintaining a healthy weight.

3. **Thyroid Hormones (T3 and T4):**

   - *Function:* The thyroid hormones T3 (triiodothyronine) and T4 (thyroxine) play a key role in regulating metabolism. They influence the rate at which the body converts food into energy.

   - *Weight Regulation:* Imbalances in thyroid function can result in metabolic changes, affecting weight. Hypothyroidism (underactive thyroid) can lead to weight gain, while hyperthyroidism (overactive thyroid) may cause weight loss. Maintaining thyroid health is vital for proper weight management.

Balancing Hormones for Optimal Health

Achieving and maintaining optimal health involves promoting a harmonious balance of hormones within the body. Hormones act as messengers, influencing various physiological processes, and their equilibrium is crucial for overall well-being. Here are key strategies to balance hormones for optimal health:

1. **Nutrient-Dense Diet:**

    - *Importance:* Nutrient-rich foods provide essential vitamins and minerals necessary for hormone production and regulation.

    - *Recommendations:* Include a variety of fruits, vegetables, whole grains, lean proteins, and healthy fats in your diet. Avoid excessive consumption of processed foods and refined sugars, as they can contribute to hormonal imbalances.

2. **Regular Physical Activity:**

    - *Importance:* Exercise helps regulate hormones, including insulin and cortisol, and contributes to overall metabolic health.

- *Recommendations:* Engage in a mix of cardiovascular exercises, strength training, and flexibility exercises. Aim for at least 150 minutes of moderate-intensity exercise per week.

3. **Adequate Sleep:**

   - *Importance:* Quality sleep is essential for hormonal balance, including cortisol, growth hormone, and leptin.

   - *Recommendations:* Aim for 7-9 hours of uninterrupted sleep per night. Create a sleep-friendly environment and establish a consistent sleep schedule.

4. **Stress Management:**

   - *Importance:* Chronic stress can lead to elevated cortisol levels, impacting hormonal balance and overall health.

   - *Recommendations:* Incorporate stress-reducing practices such as meditation, deep breathing exercises, yoga, or mindfulness into your daily routine.

5. **Hydration:**

   - *Importance:* Water is crucial for various bodily functions, including hormone transportation and balance.

- *Recommendations:* Stay adequately hydrated by drinking water throughout the day. Limit excessive caffeine and alcohol intake, as they can affect hydration and hormone levels.

6. **Maintain a Healthy Weight:**

   - *Importance:* Excess body weight, especially abdominal fat, can contribute to hormonal imbalances.

   - *Recommendations:* Adopt a balanced diet and engage in regular physical activity to achieve and maintain a healthy weight.

7. **Limit Exposure to Endocrine Disruptors:**

   - *Importance:* Certain chemicals in everyday products can interfere with hormone production and function.

   - *Recommendations:* Choose natural and organic products when possible, and be mindful of potential endocrine disruptors in household items, personal care products, and food packaging.

8. **Regular Health Check-ups:**

- *Importance:* Regular medical check-ups can help identify and address hormonal imbalances or underlying health conditions.

- *Recommendations:* Schedule routine visits with healthcare professionals for comprehensive health assessments, including hormone levels if necessary.

The Revolutionary Diet Blueprint
A Whole-Foods Approach to Nutritional Wellness

Embracing a whole-foods approach to nutrition is a fundamental step towards achieving and maintaining optimal health. This approach involves prioritizing nutrient-dense, minimally processed foods that provide essential vitamins, minerals, and other beneficial compounds. Here's a guide to adopting a whole-foods approach for nutritional wellness:

1. **Fruits and Vegetables:**

   - *Importance:* Rich in vitamins, minerals, fiber, and antioxidants, fruits and vegetables support overall health and contribute to disease prevention.

   - *Incorporation:* Aim to fill half your plate with a variety of colorful fruits and vegetables. Include both raw and cooked options for a diverse nutrient profile.

2. **Whole Grains:**

   - *Importance:* Whole grains, such as brown rice, quinoa, and oats, offer fiber, vitamins, and minerals that refined grains lack.

- *Incorporation:* Choose whole grains over refined counterparts. Options include whole-grain bread, brown rice, whole oats, and quinoa.

3. **Lean Proteins:**

- *Importance:* Protein is crucial for muscle maintenance, immune function, and overall cellular health.

- *Incorporation:* Include lean protein sources like poultry, fish, beans, lentils, tofu, and nuts in your meals. Limit processed and red meats.

4. **Healthy Fats:**

- *Importance:* Essential for brain health, hormone production, and nutrient absorption.

- *Incorporation:* Choose sources of healthy fats, such as avocados, nuts, seeds, olive oil, and fatty fish like salmon.

5. **Dairy or Dairy Alternatives:**

   - *Importance:* A source of calcium, vitamin D, and protein for bone health and overall well-being.

   - *Incorporation:* Opt for low-fat or non-fat dairy products, or choose dairy alternatives like almond milk or soy milk fortified with essential nutrients.

6. **Herbs and Spices:**

   - *Importance:* Besides adding flavor without extra calories or sodium, many herbs and spices offer potential health benefits.

   - *Incorporation:* Experiment with herbs and spices like basil, turmeric, garlic, and ginger to enhance the taste of your dishes.

7. **Minimize Processed Foods:**

   - *Importance:* Processed foods often contain added sugars, unhealthy fats, and artificial additives, contributing to various health issues.

   - *Incorporation:* Limit the consumption of processed snacks, sugary beverages, and pre-packaged meals. Opt for homemade alternatives using whole ingredients.

8. Hydration:

- *Importance:* Water is essential for digestion, nutrient absorption, and overall bodily functions.

- *Incorporation:* Drink plenty of water throughout the day. Herbal teas and infused water are refreshing alternatives.

9. Mindful Eating:

- *Importance:* Paying attention to hunger and fullness cues promotes a healthier relationship with food.

- *Incorporation:* Eat slowly, savor each bite, and listen to your body's signals. Avoid distractions, such as screens, during meals.

Hormones play a crucial role in regulating various physiological functions within the body, including metabolism and weight management. Understanding how hormones impact weight can provide valuable insights into designing an effective approach to weight loss and overall health. Here's a brief overview of key hormones and their influence on weight:

1. **Insulin:**

    - *Role:* Regulates blood sugar levels by facilitating the absorption of glucose into cells.

    - *Impact on Weight:* High insulin levels, often associated with refined carbohydrate consumption, can lead to increased fat storage. Balancing insulin is essential for effective weight management.

2. **Leptin:**

    - *Role:* Produced by fat cells, leptin signals to the brain when the body has had enough to eat, promoting feelings of fullness.

    - *Impact on Weight:* Leptin resistance can occur, where the brain doesn't respond adequately to leptin signals, leading to overeating and weight gain.

3. **Ghrelin:**

   - *Role:* Known as the "hunger hormone," ghrelin stimulates appetite and promotes the intake of food.

   - *Impact on Weight:* Imbalances in ghrelin levels can result in increased hunger, making it challenging to maintain a healthy weight.

4. **Cortisol:**

   - *Role:* Released in response to stress, cortisol helps the body cope with challenges.

   - *Impact on Weight:* Chronic stress and elevated cortisol levels can lead to increased abdominal fat storage and cravings for unhealthy foods.

5. **Thyroid Hormones (T3 and T4):**

   - *Role:* Regulate metabolism by influencing the rate at which the body burns calories.

   - *Impact on Weight:* Imbalances in thyroid hormones can lead to weight fluctuations, fatigue, and changes in energy levels.

6. **Estrogen and Testosterone:**

   - *Role:* Besides their reproductive functions, these hormones influence body composition and fat distribution.

   - *Impact on Weight:* Hormonal imbalances, such as low estrogen in women or low testosterone in men, can contribute to weight gain and difficulties in losing weight.

7. **Adiponectin:**

   - *Role:* Released by fat cells, adiponectin helps regulate glucose levels and fatty acid breakdown.

   - *Impact on Weight:* Higher levels of adiponectin are associated with better insulin sensitivity and a lower risk of obesity-related diseases.

Understanding the intricate interplay of these hormones is essential for tailoring a diet and lifestyle that supports hormonal balance, promoting effective weight management and overall well-being.

The Role of Insulin, Cortisol, and Thyroid Hormones in Weight Regulation

1. **Insulin:**

   - *Function:* Insulin is a hormone produced by the pancreas that plays a pivotal role in regulating blood sugar levels. It facilitates the uptake of glucose by cells for energy or storage.

   - *Weight Regulation:* High insulin levels, often triggered by the consumption of refined carbohydrates and sugary foods, promote fat storage. Controlling insulin spikes through a balanced diet can contribute to weight management.

2. **Cortisol:**

   - *Function:* Cortisol, often referred to as the stress hormone, is produced by the adrenal glands in response to stress. It helps the body cope with challenges by mobilizing energy reserves.

   - *Weight Regulation:* Chronic stress and consistently elevated cortisol levels can lead to increased abdominal fat storage. Managing stress through relaxation techniques and adequate sleep is crucial for maintaining a healthy wcight.

3. **Thyroid Hormones (T3 and T4):**

- *Function:* The thyroid hormones T3 (triiodothyronine) and T4 (thyroxine) play a key role in regulating metabolism. They influence the rate at which the body converts food into energy.

- *Weight Regulation:* Imbalances in thyroid function can result in metabolic changes, affecting weight. Hypothyroidism (underactive thyroid) can lead to weight gain, while hyperthyroidism (overactive thyroid) may cause weight loss. Maintaining thyroid health is vital for proper weight management.

Optimizing Fat Loss with Intermittent Fasting Strategies

Intermittent fasting (IF) is an eating pattern that cycles between periods of eating and fasting, and it has gained popularity for its potential benefits in fat loss and overall health. Here are some effective intermittent fasting strategies to optimize fat loss:

1. **16/8 Method (Time-Restricted Eating):**

   - *Overview:* This method involves fasting for 16 hours each day and restricting eating to an 8-hour window.

   - *Implementation:* For example, if you choose an eating window from 12:00 pm to 8:00 pm, you would fast from 8:00 pm to 12:00 pm the next day.

2. **5:2 Diet (Modified Fasting):**

   - *Overview:* This approach involves regular eating for five days a week and significantly reducing calorie intake (around 500-600 calories) on two non-consecutive days.

   - *Implementation:* For instance, on fasting days, you might consume a small, nutrient-dense meal for breakfast and dinner.

3. **Eat-Stop-Eat:**

- *Overview:* This method includes 24-hour fasting once or twice a week.

- *Implementation:* For example, if you finish dinner at 7:00 pm, you would fast until the next day at 7:00 pm. Water, herbal tea, and black coffee are typically allowed during the fasting period.

4. **Alternate-Day Fasting:**

- *Overview:* This involves alternating between days of regular eating and days of either very low-calorie intake or complete fasting.

- *Implementation:* On fasting days, calorie intake is reduced, while regular meals are consumed on non-fasting days.

5. **Warrior Diet:**

- *Overview:* This approach involves consuming small amounts of raw fruits and vegetables during the day and having one large meal at night within a 4-hour eating window.

- *Implementation:* Fast for 20 hours and eat during the remaining 4-hour window, typically in the evening.

6. **Spontaneous Meal Skipping:**

   - *Overview:* This less structured approach involves occasional meal skipping based on personal preference or schedule.

   - *Implementation:* Skip meals when not hungry or when it fits into your daily routine. Listen to your body's hunger cues.

Tips for Successful Intermittent Fasting:

1. **Stay Hydrated:** Drink water, herbal tea, and black coffee during fasting periods to stay hydrated and curb hunger.

2. **Choose Nutrient-Dense Foods:** Opt for whole, nutrient-dense foods during eating windows to meet essential nutritional needs.

3. **Be Consistent:** Choose an intermittent fasting strategy that aligns with your lifestyle and be consistent to see long-term benefits.

4. **Monitor Hunger Levels:** Pay attention to your body's hunger cues and adjust your fasting window or meal sizes accordingly.

5. **Exercise Smart:** Consider scheduling workouts during eating windows to support performance and recovery.

6. **Consult a Professional:** Before starting any intermittent fasting regimen, consult with a healthcare professional or nutritionist, especially if you have underlying health conditions.

20 Delicious Recipes for Fat Loss and Hormonal Harmony

. Spicy Avocado and Chickpea Salad:

- **Ingredients:**

    - Ripe avocados
    - Canned chickpeas
    - Cherry tomatoes
    - Red onion
    - Fresh cilantro
    - Lime juice
    - Olive oil
    - Salt and pepper

Instructions:

1. Dice avocados, tomatoes, and red onion.
2. Rinse chickpeas and combine with vegetables.
3. Mix in chopped cilantro.
4. Dress with lime juice, olive oil, salt, and pepper.

2. Turmeric-Infused Cauliflower Rice Bowl:

Ingredients:

- Cauliflower
- Turmeric
- Mixed vegetables (broccoli, bell peppers, carrots)
- Lean protein (chicken, tofu)
- Olive oil
- Garlic
- Ginger
- Soy sauce

Instructions:

1. Grate cauliflower into rice-sized pieces.
2. Sauté garlic and ginger in olive oil.
3. Add cauliflower rice and turmeric, cook until tender.
4. Stir in mixed vegetables and protein.
5. Season with soy sauce.

3. Salmon and Asparagus Parcels:

Ingredients:

- Salmon fillets
- Fresh asparagus spears
- Lemon slices
- Dill
- Olive oil
- Garlic
- Salt and pepper

Instructions:

1. Place salmon on foil.
2. Arrange asparagus around salmon.
3. Drizzle with olive oil, sprinkle with minced garlic, dill, salt, and pepper.
4. Seal parcels and bake until salmon is cooked.

4. Mango Tango Smoothie Bowl:

Ingredients:

- Frozen mango
- Greek yogurt
- Spinach
- Almond milk
- Chia seeds
- Toppings: sliced strawberries, coconut flakes, and granola.

Instructions:

1. Blend mango, yogurt, spinach, and almond milk until smooth.
2. Pour into a bowl, top with chia seeds, strawberries, coconut, and granola.

5. Lemon Garlic Herb Chicken Skewers:

Ingredients:

- Chicken breast chunks
- Lemon juice
- Garlic
- Fresh herbs (rosemary, thyme)
- Olive oil
- Salt and pepper

Instructions:

1. Marinate chicken in lemon juice, minced garlic, herbs, olive oil, salt, and pepper.
2. Skewer and grill until cooked.

6. Quinoa and Black Bean Stuffed Peppers:

Ingredients:

- Bell peppers
- Quinoa
- Black beans
- Corn

- Diced tomatoes

- Cumin, chili powder, and paprika

- Shredded cheese (optional)

Instructions:

1. Cook quinoa according to package instructions.

2. Mix quinoa with black beans, corn, diced tomatoes, and spices.

3. Stuff bell peppers, sprinkle with cheese, and bake until peppers are tender.

7. Green Goddess Detox Soup:

Ingredients:

- Broccoli

- Spinach

- Kale

- Celery

- Vegetable broth

- Garlic

- Lemon juice

- Fresh herbs (parsley, cilantro)

Instructions:

1. Sauté garlic in olive oil, add chopped vegetables.

2. Pour in vegetable broth, simmer until veggies are tender.

3. Blend the soup, add lemon juice and herbs before serving.

8. Berry Blast Chia Pudding:

Ingredients:

- Chia seeds

- Almond milk

- Mixed berries (strawberries, blueberries, raspberries)

- Vanilla extract

- Maple syrup (optional)

Instructions:

1. Mix chia seeds with almond milk, vanilla extract, and sweeten with maple syrup if desired.

2. Refrigerate overnight.

3. Top with mixed berries before serving.

9. Grilled Zucchini and Eggplant Roll-Ups:

Ingredients:

- Zucchini
- Eggplant
- Ricotta cheese
- Spinach
- Tomato sauce
- Italian seasoning
- Olive oil

Instructions:

1. Slice zucchini and eggplant thinly.
2. Grill until tender.
3. Spread ricotta on slices, add spinach, roll up, and bake with tomato sauce.

10. *Greek Yogurt and Berry Parfait:*

Ingredients:

- Greek yogurt
- Mixed berries
- Honey
- Granola

Instructions:

1. Layer Greek yogurt, berries, and granola in a glass.
2. Drizzle with honey.
3. Repeat the layers and enjoy this delightful parfait.

11. *Sesame Ginger Tofu Stir-Fry:*

Ingredients:

- Firm tofu
- Mixed vegetables (broccoli, bell peppers, snap peas)
- Soy sauce
- Sesame oil
- Ginger
- Garlic

- Green onions

- Sesame seeds

Instructions:

1. Press and cube tofu.

2. Sauté tofu with ginger, garlic, and vegetables.

3. Stir in soy sauce and sesame oil.

4. Garnish with green onions and sesame seeds.

12. Cucumber and Mint Infused Water:

Ingredients:

- Cucumber slices

- Fresh mint leaves

- Water

Instructions:

1. Combine cucumber slices and mint leaves in water.

2. Refrigerate for a refreshing, hydrating beverage.

13. Sweet Potato and Kale Hash:

Ingredients:

- Sweet potatoes
- Kale
- Red onion
- Olive oil
- Paprika
- Garlic powder
- Poached egg (optional)

Instructions:

1. Dice sweet potatoes and sauté with kale and red onion in olive oil.
2. Season with paprika and garlic powder.
3. Top with a poached egg if desired.

14. Almond Butter and Banana Overnight Oats:

Ingredients:

- Rolled oats
- Almond milk
- Almond butter

- Banana slices
- Chia seeds
- Honey (optional)

Instructions:

1. Mix oats, almond milk, almond butter, and chia seeds.
2. Layer with banana slices in a jar.
3. Refrigerate overnight and drizzle with honey before serving.

15. Garlic and Rosemary Roasted Sweet Potatoes:

Ingredients:

- Sweet potatoes
- Olive oil
- Garlic
- Fresh rosemary
- Salt and pepper

Instructions:

1. Toss sweet potato chunks with olive oil, minced garlic, and chopped rosemary.

2. Roast until golden and sprinkle with salt and pepper.

16. Spinach and Feta Stuffed Chicken Breast:

Ingredients:

- Chicken breasts
- Fresh spinach
- Feta cheese
- Garlic
- Olive oil
- Lemon juice
- Salt and pepper

Instructions:

1. Butterfly chicken breasts.

2. Sauté spinach and garlic in olive oil until wilted.

3. Stuff chicken with spinach mixture and feta.

4. Bake until chicken is cooked, and finish with a squeeze of lemon juice.

17. Berry Spinach Salad with Balsamic Vinaigrette

Ingredients:

- Baby spinach
- Mixed berries (strawberries, blueberries, raspberries)
- Feta cheese
- Candied pecans
- Balsamic vinaigrette dressing

Instructions:

1. Toss spinach with berries, feta, and candied pecans.

2. Drizzle with balsamic vinaigrette.

18. Cabbage and Carrot Slaw with Avocado Dressing:

- **Ingredients:**

  - Shredded cabbage

  - Grated carrots

  - Red bell pepper

  - Avocado

  - Lime juice

  - Cilantro

  - Salt and pepper

Instructions:

1. Mix cabbage, carrots, and bell pepper.

2. Blend avocado, lime juice, cilantro, salt, and pepper for the dressing.

3. Toss the slaw with the avocado dressing.

19. Pesto Zoodles with Cherry Tomatoes:

Ingredients:

- Zucchini noodles (zoodles)
- Cherry tomatoes
- Pesto sauce
- Parmesan cheese
- Pine nuts

Instructions:

1. Sauté zoodles and cherry tomatoes in a pan.
2. Toss with pesto sauce.
3. Top with Parmesan cheese and pine nuts.

20. Blueberry Almond Protein Smoothie:

Ingredients:

- Blueberries (fresh or frozen)
- Almond milk
- Greek yogurt
- Almond butter
- Protein powder
- Ice cubes

Instructions:

1. Blend blueberries, almond milk, Greek yogurt, almond butter, protein powder, and ice cubes until smooth.

Incorporating Exercise for Maximum Results

The Role of Exercise in Hormonal Balance

Exercise plays a pivotal role in maintaining hormonal balance, influencing various physiological processes within the body. Regular physical activity can positively impact hormones, promoting overall well-being. Here's an overview of how exercise contributes to hormonal balance:

1. **Endorphin Release:**

   - *Function:* Endorphins are neurotransmitters that act as natural mood elevators and pain relievers.

   - *Exercise Impact:* Physical activity, especially aerobic exercise, stimulates the release of endorphins, contributing to a positive mood and reduced stress.

2. **Insulin Sensitivity:**

   - *Function:* Insulin regulates blood sugar levels by facilitating glucose absorption into cells.

- *Exercise Impact:* Regular exercise improves insulin sensitivity, helping to regulate blood sugar and reduce the risk of insulin resistance.

3. **Cortisol Regulation:**

   - *Function:* Cortisol, the stress hormone, influences metabolism, immune function, and blood pressure.

   - *Exercise Impact:* Moderate-intensity exercise helps regulate cortisol levels, reducing chronic stress and its potential negative effects on hormonal balance.

4. **Growth Hormone Production:**

   - *Function:* Growth hormone is essential for growth, cell repair, and metabolism.

   - *Exercise Impact:* High-intensity activities, such as strength training and interval training, stimulate the production of growth hormone, promoting muscle development and fat metabolism.

5. **Thyroid Hormones:**

- *Function:* Thyroid hormones (T3 and T4) influence metabolism and energy expenditure.

- *Exercise Impact:* Regular exercise contributes to the proper functioning of the thyroid gland, supporting optimal thyroid hormone levels.

6. **Sex Hormones:**

   - *Function:* Sex hormones, including estrogen and testosterone, play crucial roles in reproductive health and overall well-being.

   - *Exercise Impact:* Moderate exercise can positively influence sex hormone balance, contributing to reproductive health and bone density.

7. **Leptin and Ghrelin Regulation:**

   - *Function:* Leptin signals satiety, while ghrelin stimulates appetite.

   - *Exercise Impact:* Physical activity helps regulate leptin and ghrelin levels, promoting a healthy appetite and weight management.

8. **Anti-Inflammatory Effects:**

- *Function:* Chronic inflammation is linked to various health issues.

- *Exercise Impact:* Regular exercise has anti-inflammatory effects, reducing the risk of inflammatory-related hormonal imbalances.

Tips for Hormonally Balanced Exercise:

1. **Include a Mix of Activities:** Combine aerobic exercises, strength training, and flexibility exercises for comprehensive hormonal benefits.

2. **Consistency is Key:** Regular, consistent exercise is more effective in maintaining hormonal balance than sporadic intense workouts.

3. **Adequate Recovery:** Allow time for rest and recovery to prevent overtraining, which can negatively impact hormones.

4. **Manage Stress:** Incorporate stress-reducing activities like meditation and yoga to complement your exercise routine.

5. **Customize for Individual Needs:** Consider individual factors such as age, fitness level,

and health status when planning an exercise routine.

High-Intensity Interval Training (HIIT) for Effective Fat Loss

High-Intensity Interval Training (HIIT) has gained popularity as a powerful and time-efficient workout method for fat loss. This form of exercise alternates between short bursts of intense activity and periods of rest or lower-intensity exercise. Here's how HIIT contributes to fat loss and some guidelines for incorporating it into your fitness routine:

How HIIT Promotes Fat Loss:

1. **Increased Caloric Expenditure:**

   - *Mechanism:* HIIT engages multiple muscle groups intensely, leading to a higher calorie burn during and after the workout (known as the afterburn effect or excess post-exercise oxygen consumption - EPOC).

   - *Result:* This increased caloric expenditure contributes to overall fat loss.

2. **Improved Metabolism:**

   - *Mechanism:* HIIT enhances metabolic rate, promoting the body's ability to burn calories efficiently.

   - *Result:* A more efficient metabolism supports fat loss, even during periods of rest.

3. **Elevated Fat Oxidation:**

   - *Mechanism:* HIIT encourages the body to use fat as a fuel source during and after exercise.

   - *Result:* This shift toward fat oxidation contributes to a reduction in body fat over time.

4. **Enhanced Insulin Sensitivity:**

   - *Mechanism:* HIIT improves insulin sensitivity, helping the body regulate blood sugar more effectively.

   - *Result:* Better insulin sensitivity reduces the likelihood of excess glucose being stored as fat.

5. **Appetite Regulation:**

   - *Mechanism:* HIIT has been associated with appetite regulation hormones, potentially reducing feelings of hunger post-exercise.

- *Result:* Controlled appetite can support healthier food choices and calorie intake.

Guidelines for HIIT Sessions:

1. **Choose Your Exercises:**

   - *Examples:* Sprinting, cycling, jumping jacks, burpees, and high knees.

   - *Variety:* Mix cardio and bodyweight exercises for a well-rounded workout.

2. **Intensity and Duration:**

   - *Work-Interval:* 20-60 seconds of maximum effort.

   - *Rest-Interval:* 20-60 seconds to allow for recovery.

   - *Repetition:* Repeat the cycle for 15-30 minutes.

3. **Frequency:**

   - *Start Gradually:* Begin with 1-2 sessions per week.

- *Progression:* Gradually increase frequency as your fitness level improves.

4. **Warm-Up and Cool Down:**

   - *Warm-Up:* 5-10 minutes of light cardio and dynamic stretches.

   - *Cool Down:* 5-10 minutes of static stretching to enhance flexibility and reduce muscle soreness.

5. **Listen to Your Body:**

   - *Intensity:* Tailor the intensity to your fitness level.

   - *Rest as Needed:* Take longer rest intervals if necessary, especially for beginners.

6. **Combine with Other Exercises:**

   - *Complement:* Incorporate HIIT with other forms of exercise like strength training and steady-state cardio for a balanced fitness routine.

7. **Consult a Professional:**

   - *Individualization:* If you have pre-existing health conditions, consult with a fitness professional or healthcare provider to tailor HIIT to your specific needs.

Strength Training for Hormonal Optimization

Strength training, also known as resistance or weight training, is a powerful exercise modality with significant implications for hormonal optimization. This form of exercise involves working against resistance to improve muscular strength and endurance. Here's how strength training positively influences hormones and contributes to overall hormonal balance:

1. Growth Hormone Production:

- *Mechanism:* Intense strength training, particularly compound movements like squats and deadlifts, stimulates the release of growth hormone.

- *Result:* Increased growth hormone levels aid in muscle development, fat metabolism, and overall cellular repair.

2. Testosterone Regulation:

- *Mechanism:* Strength training, especially with heavy loads, can lead to a transient increase in testosterone levels.

- *Result:* Enhanced testosterone levels support muscle growth, bone density, and overall vitality.

3. Insulin Sensitivity:

- *Mechanism:* Regular strength training improves insulin sensitivity, facilitating better blood sugar regulation.

- *Result:* Improved insulin sensitivity contributes to reduced fat storage and a lowered risk of insulin resistance.

4. Cortisol Management:

- *Mechanism:* While strength training can temporarily increase cortisol levels during the session, it helps manage overall cortisol balance over the long term.

- *Result:* Proper cortisol balance supports stress management and prevents chronic cortisol elevation, which can lead to hormonal imbalances.

5. Thyroid Function:

- *Mechanism:* Strength training positively influences thyroid hormones, supporting overall metabolic function.

- *Result:* A well-functioning thyroid contributes to energy production and efficient calorie utilization.

6. Metabolic Rate Enhancement:

- *Mechanism:* Muscle is metabolically active tissue, and strength training helps increase lean muscle mass.

- *Result:* A higher muscle-to-fat ratio enhances the resting metabolic rate, promoting fat loss and weight management.

7. Leptin and Ghrelin Regulation:

- *Mechanism:* Strength training can influence appetite-regulating hormones such as leptin and ghrelin.

- *Result:* Improved hormonal regulation of appetite supports healthier eating habits and weight management.

8. Bone Density Improvement:

- *Mechanism:* Weight-bearing exercises involved in strength training stimulate bone formation.

- *Result:* Increased bone density reduces the risk of osteoporosis, especially important for hormonal health in women.

1. **Include Compound Exercises:**

   - *Examples:* Squats, deadlifts, bench press, and overhead press.

   - *Rationale:* Compound exercises engage multiple muscle groups, maximizing hormonal responses.

2. **Progressive Overload:**

   - *Principle:* Gradually increase resistance or intensity to challenge the muscles.

   - *Rationale:* Progressive overload is essential for continued strength gains and hormonal benefits.

3. **Balanced Routine:**

   - *Incorporate:* Include a mix of exercises targeting different muscle groups.

   - *Rationale:* Balanced training prevents muscle imbalances and supports overall strength development.

4. **Rest and Recovery:**

- *Schedule:* Allow at least 48 hours of rest between strength training sessions for specific muscle groups.

- *Rationale:* Adequate recovery is crucial for muscle repair and hormonal balance.

5. **Form and Technique:**

   - *Focus:* Prioritize proper form over heavy weights.

   - *Rationale:* Correct form minimizes the risk of injury and maximizes the effectiveness of each exercise.

6. **Consistency:**

   - *Frequency:* Aim for at least two to three strength training sessions per week.

   - *Rationale:* Consistent training is key to reaping long-term hormonal benefits.

7. **Individualization:**

   - *Consultation:* Consider seeking guidance from a fitness professional, especially if you have specific health concerns or conditions.

- *Rationale:* Tailoring a strength training program to individual needs ensures safety and effectiveness.

Mind-Body Connection

Effective Stress Management Techniques

In the modern world, stress has become a common part of daily life, impacting both physical and mental well-being. Employing effective stress management techniques is essential for maintaining a healthy balance and preventing long-term negative consequences. Here are various strategies to help manage and reduce stress:

1. **Deep Breathing and Relaxation:**

   - *Technique:* Practice deep, diaphragmatic breathing. Inhale deeply through your nose, hold for a few seconds, and exhale slowly through your mouth. Combine this with progressive muscle relaxation, starting from your toes and working your way up.

2. **Mindfulness Meditation:**

   - *Technique:* Engage in mindfulness or meditation practices. Focus on your breath or a specific point of attention, allowing yourself to be present in the moment without judgment. Apps and guided sessions can be helpful.

3. **Regular Exercise:**

   - *Activity:* Engage in regular physical activity, such as walking, jogging, or yoga.

   - *Rationale:* Exercise releases endorphins, reduces cortisol levels, and promotes overall well-being.

4. **Time Management:**

   - *Strategy:* Prioritize tasks and break them into smaller, manageable steps.

   - *Rationale:* Organizing your time effectively can help prevent feelings of overwhelm and reduce stress.

5. **Healthy Lifestyle Choices:**

   - *Habits:* Adopt a balanced diet, ensure adequate sleep, and limit caffeine and alcohol intake.

   - *Rationale:* A healthy lifestyle contributes to overall resilience and the body's ability to cope with stress.

6. **Social Support:**

- *Action:* Connect with friends, family, or support groups.

- *Rationale:* Sharing your feelings and experiences can provide emotional support and perspective.

7. **Positive Affirmations:**

- *Practice:* Use positive affirmations to counter negative thoughts.

- *Rationale:* Shifting your mindset towards positivity can help manage stress.

8. **Journaling:**

- *Method:* Write down your thoughts and feelings in a journal.

- *Rationale:* Journaling can provide an outlet for self-reflection and emotional expression.

9. **Hobbies and Creative Outlets:**

- *Engagement:* Pursue activities you enjoy, whether it's art, music, or gardening.

- *Rationale:* Engaging in hobbies can be a therapeutic way to redirect focus and alleviate stress.

10. **Cognitive Behavioral Therapy (CBT):**

    - *Approach:* Work with a therapist to identify and change negative thought patterns.

    - *Rationale:* CBT provides effective tools for managing stress by addressing thought processes and behaviors.

11. **Nature and Green Spaces:**

    - *Activity:* Spend time in nature, whether it's a walk in the park or gardening.

    - *Rationale:* Nature has a calming effect and promotes relaxation.

12. **Limiting Technology Use:**

    - *Practice:* Set boundaries for screen time and social media.

    - *Rationale:* Excessive technology use can contribute to stress; taking breaks can be beneficial.

13. **Humor and Laughter:**

- *Practice:* Find humor in everyday situations, watch a funny movie, or spend time with people who make you laugh.

- *Rationale:* Laughter releases endorphins and provides a natural stress relief.

14. **Learn to Say No:**

- *Skill:* Establish boundaries and feel comfortable saying no when necessary.

- *Rationale:* Avoiding overcommitment helps prevent stress from overwhelming you.

15. **Professional Support:**

- *Resource:* Seek help from a mental health professional when needed.

- *Rationale:* Therapists can provide coping strategies and support for managing stress.

Adequate Sleep and Its Impact on Hormones

Quality sleep is crucial for overall health, and it plays a significant role in hormonal regulation. Sleep affects various hormones that influence metabolism, stress, appetite, and overall well-being. Here's an overview of how adequate sleep impacts key hormones:

1. Cortisol Regulation:

- *Role:* Cortisol, the stress hormone, helps regulate the sleep-wake cycle.

- *Impact of Sleep:* Adequate sleep contributes to a normal cortisol rhythm, ensuring it peaks in the early morning and decreases at night. Poor sleep can lead to elevated cortisol levels, potentially causing stress-related issues.

2. Growth Hormone Release:

- *Role:* Growth hormone is essential for growth, cell repair, and metabolism.

- *Impact of Sleep:* The majority of growth hormone is released during deep sleep (slow-wave sleep). Consistent, good-quality sleep supports optimal growth hormone production, promoting muscle repair and fat metabolism.

3. Leptin and Ghrelin Balance:

- *Role:* Leptin signals satiety, while ghrelin stimulates appetite.

- *Impact of Sleep:* Inadequate sleep disrupts the balance between leptin and ghrelin, leading to increased hunger and potential weight gain. A well-rested individual is more likely to maintain a healthy appetite.

4. Insulin Sensitivity:

- *Role:* Insulin regulates blood sugar levels.

- *Impact of Sleep:* Insufficient sleep can reduce insulin sensitivity, leading to impaired glucose metabolism. This increases the risk of insulin resistance and Type 2 diabetes.

5. Melatonin Production:

- *Role:* Melatonin is the hormone that regulates the sleep-wake cycle.

- *Impact of Sleep:* Quality sleep enhances melatonin production, promoting the natural sleep cycle. Exposure to artificial light at night or irregular sleep patterns can disrupt melatonin production, affecting sleep quality.

6. Testosterone Levels:

- *Role:* Testosterone is crucial for muscle development, bone density, and overall vitality.

- *Impact of Sleep:* Testosterone is primarily released during deep sleep. Chronic sleep deprivation or poor sleep quality can lead to decreased testosterone levels, impacting muscle health and overall energy.

7. Thyroid Hormones:

- *Role:* Thyroid hormones (T3 and T4) influence metabolism and energy expenditure.

- *Impact of Sleep:* Sleep deprivation may disrupt the production and regulation of thyroid hormones, affecting metabolic function.

8. Stress Hormone Regulation (Adrenocorticotropic Hormone - ACTH):

- *Role:* ACTH stimulates the release of cortisol.

- *Impact of Sleep:* Adequate sleep helps regulate ACTH, preventing excessive cortisol release. Chronic sleep deprivation can lead to heightened stress responses.

Tips for Improving Sleep and Hormonal Balance

1. **Consistent Sleep Schedule:**

   - *Routine:* Go to bed and wake up at the same time every day, even on weekends.

   - *Rationale:* Consistency helps regulate the body's internal clock.

2. **Create a Relaxing Bedtime Routine:**

   - *Activities:* Engage in calming activities before bedtime, such as reading or practicing relaxation techniques.

   - *Rationale:* A consistent routine signals to the body that it's time to wind down.

3. **Optimize Sleep Environment:**

   - *Factors:* Ensure a comfortable mattress, cool room temperature, and minimal light and noise.

   - *Rationale:* A conducive sleep environment enhances sleep quality.

4. **Limit Screen Time Before Bed:**

- *Recommendation:* Avoid electronic devices at least an hour before bedtime.

- *Rationale:* The blue light emitted from screens can suppress melatonin production.

5. **Mindful Eating and Hydration:**

- *Timing:* Avoid heavy meals close to bedtime and stay hydrated.

- *Rationale:* Discomfort from digestion or thirst can disrupt sleep.

6. **Regular Exercise:**

- *Timing:* Engage in regular physical activity, but avoid intense workouts close to bedtime.

- *Rationale:* Exercise promotes better sleep, but timing is essential to prevent interference with sleep onset.

7. **Manage Stress:**

- *Practices:* Incorporate stress management techniques such as meditation or deep breathing.

- *Rationale:* Reducing stress levels contributes to a more restful sleep.

8. **Limit Caffeine and Alcohol:**

   - *Recommendation:* Avoid consuming caffeine and alcohol close to bedtime.

   - *Rationale:* These substances can disrupt sleep patterns.

Mindful Eating for Hormonal Harmony

Mindful eating is a practice that involves being fully present and engaged in the act of eating. This approach not only enhances the sensory experience of food but also has positive implications for hormonal balance. Here's how mindful eating contributes to hormonal harmony:

1. Improved Insulin Sensitivity:

- *Practice:* Paying attention to the flavors and textures of food, and recognizing feelings of hunger and fullness.

- *Result:* Mindful eating can improve insulin sensitivity, aiding in better blood sugar control and reducing the risk of insulin resistance.

2. Stress Reduction:

- *Practice:* Eating without distractions, such as phones or computers, and focusing on the act of eating.

- *Result:* Reduced stress during meals can positively impact cortisol levels, promoting hormonal balance.

3. Leptin and Ghrelin Regulation:

- *Practice:* Eating slowly and savoring each bite, allowing time for the body to signal fullness.

- *Result:* Mindful eating helps regulate the balance between leptin (satiety hormone) and ghrelin (hunger hormone), supporting a healthier appetite.

4. Emotional Eating Awareness:

- *Practice:* Recognizing emotional triggers for eating and addressing them consciously.

- *Result:* Mindful eating discourages impulsive or emotionally-driven eating, promoting a more balanced relationship with food.

5. Enhanced Digestion:

- *Practice:* Chewing food thoroughly and savoring each bite.

- *Result:* Improved digestion and nutrient absorption, contributing to overall hormonal and metabolic health.

6. Ghrelin and Meal Timing:

- *Practice:* Listening to natural hunger cues and eating when genuinely hungry.

- *Result:* Mindful eating can help maintain a regular meal schedule, positively impacting ghrelin levels and preventing excessive snacking.

7. Connection Between Mind and Body:

- *Practice:* Bringing awareness to physical sensations, such as hunger and fullness.

- *Result:* A strengthened mind-body connection fosters a more intuitive approach to eating, promoting hormonal harmony.

8. Reduced Cortisol Levels:

- *Practice:* Avoiding stress-inducing behaviors while eating, such as multitasking or rushing.

- *Result:* Lowered cortisol levels during meals contribute to a calmer physiological state, supporting hormonal balance.

Tips for Incorporating Mindful Eating:

1. **Engage Your Senses:**

   - *Suggestion:* Notice the colors, textures, and aromas of your food.

   - *Rationale:* Engaging the senses enhances the eating experience and fosters mindfulness.

2. **Eat Without Distractions:**

   - *Recommendation:* Avoid using electronic devices or watching TV while eating.

   - *Rationale:* Eliminating distractions allows you to focus on the act of eating and your body's signals.

3. **Chew Thoroughly:**

- *Guideline:* Chew each bite slowly and thoroughly.

- *Rationale:* Proper chewing aids digestion and encourages a mindful approach to eating.

4. **Listen to Hunger and Fullness Cues:**

- *Reminder:* Pause and assess your level of hunger before and during meals.

- *Rationale:* Responding to natural hunger cues prevents overeating and supports hormonal balance.

5. **Mindful Portion Control:**

- *Practice:* Serve reasonable portions and be aware of portion sizes.

- *Rationale:* Mindful portion control helps prevent excessive calorie intake.

6. **Practice Gratitude:**

- *Activity:* Take a moment to express gratitude for your food.

- *Rationale:* Cultivating gratitude fosters a positive relationship with food.

7. **Identify Emotional Triggers:**

- *Step:* Recognize emotional cues that may prompt eating.

- *Rationale:* Addressing emotional triggers promotes mindful responses to food.

8. **Slow Down:**

- *Reminder:* Pace yourself during meals, and savor the experience.

- *Rationale:* Eating slowly enhances enjoyment and allows for better recognition of satiety.

CONCLUSION

As the final chapter of "Hormone Harmony: A Revolutionary Diet Plan for Igniting Fat Loss and Alleviating Hormonal Disturbances" unfolds, readers find themselves on the brink of a transformative journey's end. Dr. Amelia Roberts, the brilliant mind behind this groundbreaking approach to wellness, leaves an indelible mark on the landscape of health and vitality.The book's conclusion is not merely the end of a narrative; it marks the beginning of a new chapter in the lives of those who embraced the principles of Hormone Harmony. Through the pages, readers have discovered the intricacies of their own bodies, learning to listen to the subtle whispers of hormones and respond with tailored care. The journey wasn't always easy, but it was undeniably rewarding.In these final pages, Dr. Roberts imparts a message of empowerment. The readers are not left with a strict set of rules but rather with a newfound understanding of their bodies' unique needs. The Hormone Harmony journey, she emphasizes, is not a one-size-fits-all solution but a guide to unlocking the potential for lasting well-being.As readers close the book, they carry with them the tools to navigate the complexities of their hormonal landscapes. The journey of fat loss becomes more than a physical transformation; it becomes a holistic metamorphosis. The stories woven into each chapter, the testimonials of those who embarked on this path, serve as beacons of inspiration for others who may be standing at the crossroads of their own health.The conclusion invites reflection—a moment to celebrate the victories, acknowledge the challenges, and appreciate the resilience that comes with understanding one's body. Dr. Roberts encourages readers to continue their pursuit of Hormone Harmony, not as a destination but as an ongoing practice of self-discovery and self-care.As the final words echo in the minds of readers, a sense of empowerment lingers. The book may end, but the journey towards Hormone Harmony is a lifelong expedition—one where individuals, armed with newfound knowledge, navigate the twists and turns with confidence, embracing the vitality that comes from a harmonious balance within.